# Helenne Firr

# Eat And Lose Weight!

# Healthy Food
# For Weight Loss:
# Basic Concepts

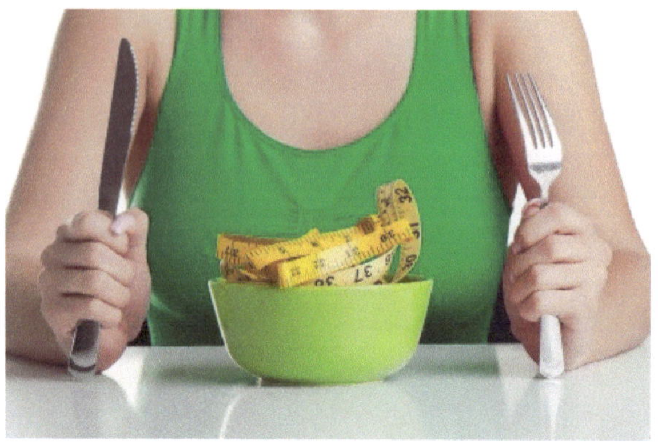

Quick weight reduction could also be harmful to your well being. The most effective weight reduction program is to drop some pounds naturally with out relying on any weight reduction tablet or drug. This text examines some on a regular basis adjustments you can simply make to your each day meals consumption that will help you obtain your ideally suited weight.

## Weight Loss Ideas: What's Your Finest Weight Loss Program?

Most individuals need quick weight reduction, however this can be harmful. Any weight reduction food plan ought to be gradual and disciplined, with out being radical or excessive.

Pure weight reduction is the most effective technique and there are some straightforward every day suggestions, that don't contain any weight reduction capsule or synthetic medicine, for a balanced weight reduction eating regimen.

It's vital that at each meal, breakfast included, you eat protein. You must cease consuming bread, pasta and different wheat and flour-based mostly merchandise.

By consuming unprocessed meals, you're giving your physique dietary gasoline. The truth is, it's best to intention at having about ninety per cent of your meals comprising of the next: lean protein, uncooked and/or steamed greens and entire grains.

**2**

Eat fruit, however eat extra greens. Solely have one piece of fruit every day, any solely eat the low sugar, excessive fibre fruits like berries, plums, pears and apples. Keep away from fruit juice as a result of it normally has method an excessive amount of sugar. Have some low fats nuts together with your piece of fruit.

You need to reduce proper again on dairy merchandise, particularly cow's milk, though you possibly can take pleasure in small helpings of fats free and low sugar yoghurt.

Alcohol and weight reduction don't go hand in hand, so strictly in the reduction of, or eradicate alcohol in your weight loss plan. Select greens and fruit as an alternative.

Use olive oil as a substitute of grocery store vegetable oils like corn, safflower and sunflower. The place potential, apply olive oil to your meals after it's cooked.

Keep away from consuming the pores and skin of fried rooster – the chicken is way extra dietary and has much less fats.

Be very aware of the quantity and kinds of fats that you're taking in along with your meals.. Unhealthy fat are in margarine and fried meals. One of the best good fat are Omega-three, present in fish and flaxseed oil. See if you happen to can eat fish no less than thrice every week, however keep in mind, no fried fish.

It's best to drink no less than eight ounces of water every day for each 20 kilos you weigh. Everytime you really feel hungry, have a glass of water.

One of the best weight reduction program is the one about which you change into very single-minded.

Hypnosis, both particular person classes with a hypno-therapist, or commonly listening to professionally recorded hypnosis classes, will also be software to think about in your weight administration plans.

Hypnotism can be certain that each your aware and un-conscious minds are aligned within the want to eat wholesome meals, to do common day by day train and to correctly handle your weight.

## Take Management Of Your Physique

## With A Wholesome Meals Food plan

The misguided consuming habits can fatally impede any weight reduction try so studying the best way to change consuming habits for weight reduction could be very essential for any dieter wishing to lose kilos. As soon as you already know the suitable meals to eat making wholesome selections to drop some weight is easy. Dropping pounds is an efficient means of enhancing your wellbeing and feeling and looking higher.

A wholesome meals eating regimen is useful for everybody. It is very important deal with your physique and when you eat effectively, you'll reap the nice advantages. A nutritious diet doesn't have to be boring! It needs to be tasty, balanced and thrilling. If you happen to get tired of a weight loss program, you'll shortly

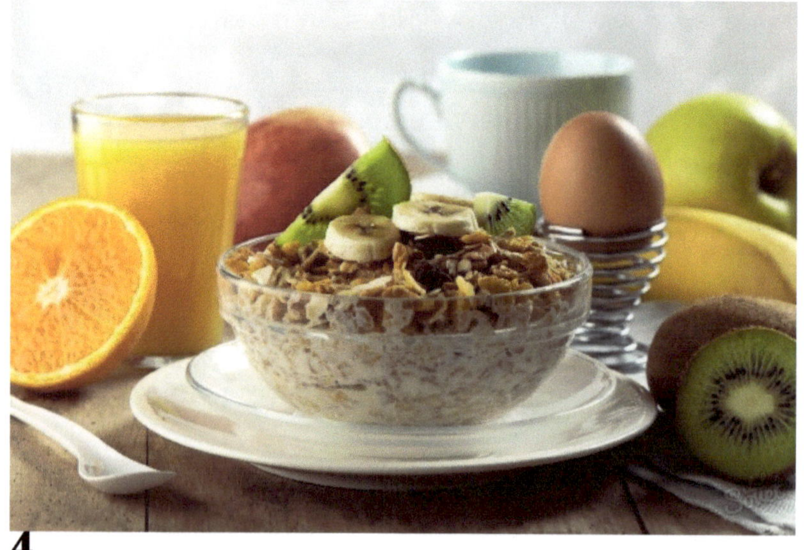

abandon it!A wholesome meals food plan is a life consuming plan fairly than a brief time period fad eating regimen (fad diets don't work as a result of your physique doesn't get all its required vitamins and you find yourself with starvation pangs and cravings).

A great wholesome meals listing is a should for folks looking for to enhance their consuming habits and begin on a food regimen of fine vitamin. Most of us are both overwhelmed by the amount of information out there on what wholesome meals are or lack the time to get organized earlier than we buy groceries. That's the reason arising with a wholesome meals record is a should.

To work greatest, the physique wants carbohydrates, proteins, fat, minerals, nutritional vitamins and liquids. A wide selection of greens, fruits, grains and proteins is important and consuming common meals slightly than only one large one is healthier for you.

Consuming properly reduces the chance of sicknesses resembling most cancers, hypertension, diabetes and coronary heart illness. A poor eating regimen may end up in weight problems, lethargy and spotty pores and skin. An excellent weight-reduction plan will enable you preserve a wholesome weight which is an enormous consider general well being.

Select meals that present a wealthy supply of most of the important vitamins wanted for optimum well being. Embrace the fruits, greens, complete grains, nuts and seeds, lean meats, fish, olive oil, herbs and spices that you simply get pleasure from and are acquainted to you and your loved ones. An occasional unique meals could also be a brand new expertise, however should you or your loved ones won't eat it, why embrace it in your record? On the subject of greens, attempt selecting from the rainbow of colours accessible to maximise selection. Purchase non-starchy greens resembling spinach, carrots, broccoli or inexperienced beans.

It's a unhealthy thought to deprive your self completely of your favourite meals so the occasional slice of chocolate cake is ok. You don't want to chop something out utterly. You'll be able to, nonetheless, make good decisions and substitute one meals alternative for an additional.Adjustments needs to be made step by step. You possibly can start by introducing extra recent fruit and greens into your food plan, and maybe swapping white processed bread for an entire grain bread.Should you usually deep fry loads of meals, attempt baking or grilling it as an alternative

Select entire grain meals as an alternative of processed grain merchandise. Strive brown rice and complete-wheat spaghetti or spinach pasta. Embrace dried beans (like kidney or pinto beans) and lentils. Select entire grain breads this implies breads that say 12 grain not simply complete wheat.Select wholesome spices and herbs to boost your meals weight loss plan. Many people should not conscious of the therapeutic powers and dietary worth of spices. Each herbs and spices are glorious antioxidants. Chili Powder, a mix of spices together with chili peppers, plus cumin, oregano, paprika, salt, and garlic powder. The well being advantages of chili powder are derived largely from the capsaicin within the purple pepper which is utilized in pores and skin lotions to cut back ache, together with that of osteoarthritis. It additionally has antioxidant and blood- thinning qualities.

## How a Diary Can Assist You Lose Weight

What if somebody instructed you that weight reduction could possibly be easy? No loopy diets, no costly appointments with nutritionists, no listing of "forbidden meals." All it's essential do is maintain a meals diary. By writing down all the pieces you eat, you may clear a path to weight reduction and make wholesome consuming a breeze. It's all about understanding serving sizes and being sincere about your each day meals consumption.

What if somebody instructed you that weight reduction might be easy? No loopy diets, no costly appointments with nutritionists, no listing of "forbidden meals". All you must do is maintain a meals diary. By writing down all the pieces you eat, you'll be able to clear a path to weight reduction and make wholesome consuming a breeze. It's all about figuring out serving sizes and being sincere about your day by day meals consumption.

All it is advisable begin are a pen and paper and these normal tips on your advisable every day weight loss plan:

Ladies:
–Seven servings of fruit and greens
–Six servings of grain merchandise
–Two to a few servings of milk and alternate options
– Two to 3 servings of meat and options

Males:
–Seven servings of fruit and greens
–Seven servings of grain merchandise
–Three servings of milk and options
–Three servings of meat and alternate options

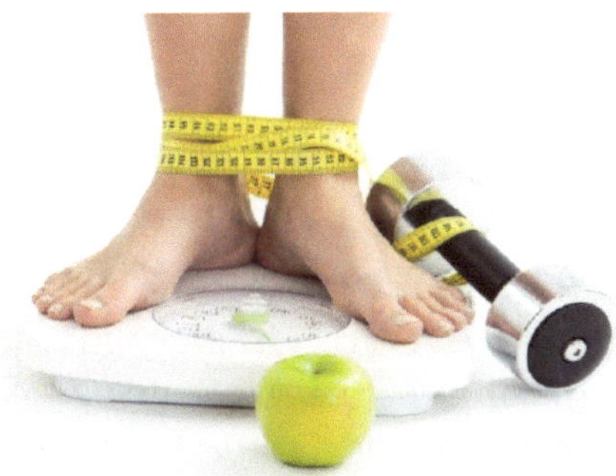

Bear in mind; conserving a meals diary is about writing down precisely what you ate and drank—not what you thought you probably did. By writing down each single nibble and the way huge the portion was, after seven days, you'll uncover every little thing you'll want to learn about constructing a profitable weight loss plan. You'll indentify whenever you overeat, or have one too many "treats." You'll additionally just remember to're getting sufficient vegatables and fruits.

At a hospital clinic in Greenwich, Connecticut, specialists have had nice success in serving to diabetic sufferers handle

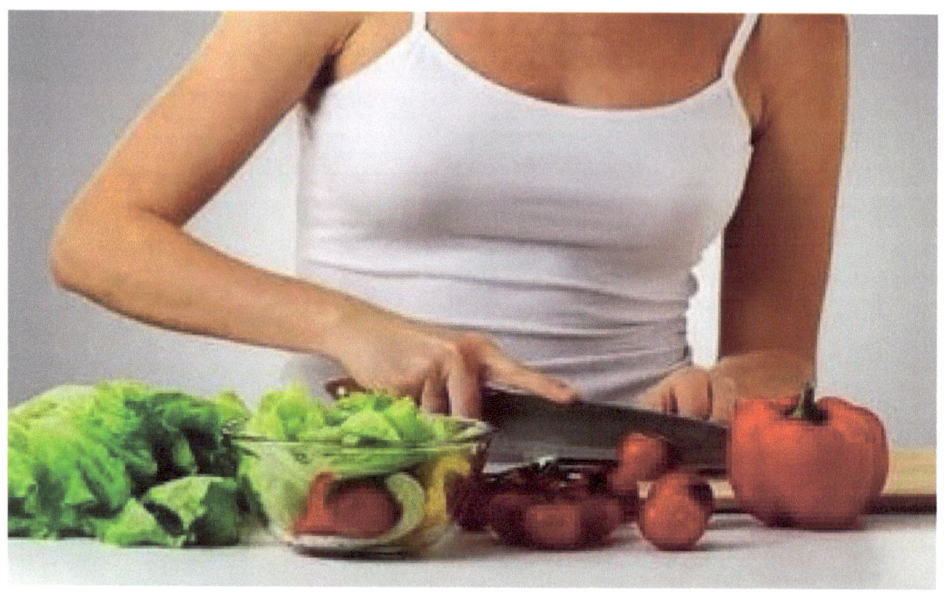

their weight. Actually, the clinic divides their sufferers into two teams: the meals diary keepers and the non-keepers. In accordance with one physician on the clinic, the individuals who preserve diaries are often very profitable and solely need assistance for about 12 weeks. However the non-diary-keepers? Sufferers who don't hold a diary generally go to the clinic for years making an attempt unsuccessfully to get additional weight off and hold it off.

Maintaining a meals diary is like train; it would all the time show you how to drop some weight in case you do it constantly. Keep in mind that dieters who maintain journals are extra profitable as a result of they're keen to acknowledge each little bit of meals they eat, and this exhibits them what number of energy they're consuming per day.

A meals diary additionally lets you keep a balanced weight loss program. In the event you're consuming 10 servings of cereals and bread and just one serving of protein each day, for instance, it's simple to see the way you could be placing on these additional kilos. Substituting extra lean protein into your food plan

**8**

will give your muscle groups extra gasoline and your abdomen much less fats to retailer.

Simply ensure you carry your diary with you all over the place. A diary will help you shed some pounds, however not in the event you don't use it!

## Wholesome Weight Loss Ought to Contain a Steadiness Weight loss plan

Weight reduction ought to be taken as an extended-time period program because the physique takes time to drop pounds in a pure method. Speedy weight reduction gained with the consumption of weight reduction weight loss supplements and meals dietary supplements deprive you of the power mandatory for each day metabolism. These dietary supplements are additionally low on important nutritional vitamins and mineral and therefore have an effect on your well being drastically. Sudden adjustments in your consuming habits put plenty of stress in your liver.

Dedication, perseverance and endurance are very essential for a wholesome weight reduction. You need to management your food regimen and train frequently until you obtain the targets set in your weight reduction program. The motivation for a wholesome weight reduction ought to come from your personal self and it's best to comply with the burden loss program with dedication.

Train is an integral a part of any weight reduction program. You must train for 30 to forty five minutes day by day. Be common in your workouts, as dropping your rhythm could be very straightforward. As soon as your make train a routine, you'll like doing it. Additionally improve your each day exercise ranges every so often. This may occasionally embody parking your automobile a bit of far-off whenever you buy groceries, beginning gardening, and many others.

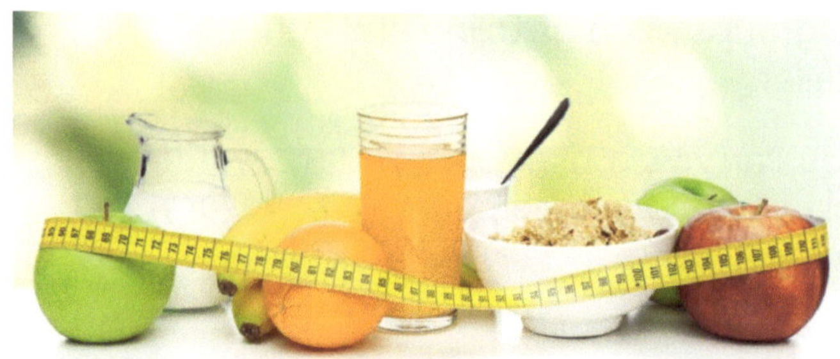

Wholesome weight reduction ought to contain a stability food plan. It is best to eat much less fat and extra proteins and carbohydrates. It is best to eat extra of fruits, greens, grains and starchy meals. You food plan shouldn't include just one meals merchandise. You need to eat quite a lot of meals gadgets. A sound well being isn't about getting ample energy for physique metabolism and is achieved by consuming varied important meals.

It's also possible to seek the advice of a registered dietician for weight reduction. Dieticians are educated and skilled in vitamin and can present you details about totally different meals gadgets, their compositions, calorific values and their advantages. You also needs to learn meals labels to get a clearer understanding of what you might be consuming. Meals which can be labeled ninety seven to 100% fats-free are good for wholesome weight reduction.

Make a sluggish begin and let your physique regulate to the brand new way of life. Don't haste and eat fat burners which will have unintended effects. You may as well select to make one to 2 adjustments in your habits each week. For instance, within the first week, you possibly can determine that you'll not eat fried meals and stroll each day throughout your lunch break. Within the second week, you'll be able to cease consuming fats wealthy dairy merchandise and begin jogging within the morning. Your physique will get enough time to react to such modifications and you'll achieve reaching wholesome weight reduction. You

**10**

shouldn't goal weight lack of greater than two kilos every week. Some folks additionally preserve a file of their weight loss plan and train. Analyze your meals habits and train ranges each week and makes essential enhancements in your weight reduction program. Enhance the amount of wholesome meals gadgets that your take and scale back the unhealthy ones each week.

You must also be common in your meals and snacks. Should you skip a meal, you can be hungry after a number of hours and your physique will demand excessive power weight loss program. You may be tempted to eat sugar-wealthy meals comparable to pastry and chocolate.

If different members in your loved ones additionally need to scale back weight, then your entire household can select to eat nutritious diet. This may scale back your entry to fats wealthy stuff and quick meals. With decreased entry, you'll be much less tempted to eat these unhealthy meals.

**In a single day Weight Loss**

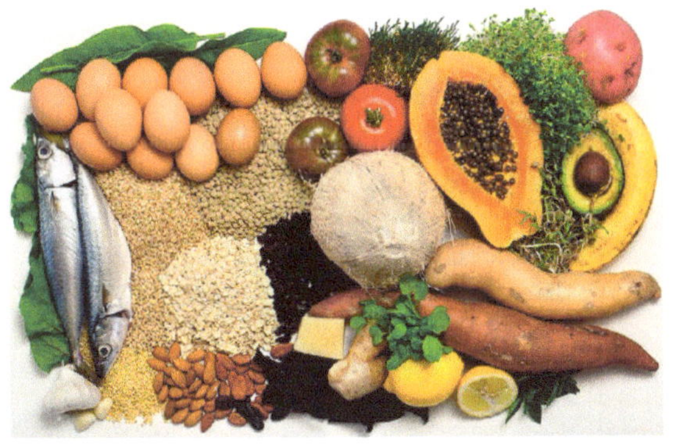

The primary and the foremost factor in the direction of a nutritious diet and life-style as a way to drop a few pounds is a wholesome diet.

Weight reduction depends upon the collection of meals that you just eat and the plans that you just lay out for train.

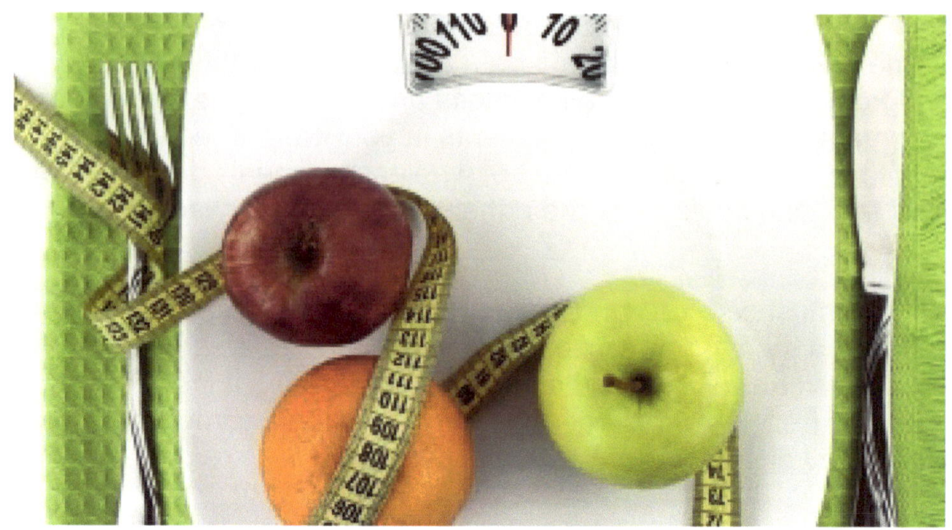

The primary and the foremost factor in the direction of a nutritious diet and way of life to be able to shed extra pounds is a wholesome diet. Weight reduction will depend on the choice of meals that you simply eat and the plans that you simply lay out for train. The principle train plan ought to embrace cardiovascular and weight coaching workouts. With this train plan, we will burn the energy and enhance the muscle mass and lose fat at a really quick tempo and then again enhance the metabolism as properly.

Weight reduction have to be achieved step by step. It's at all times greatest so that you can drop some weight at a gradual tempo. Should you shed extra pounds on a really fast tempo, it will simply go away the individual with a free pores and skin and that may solely be managed by surgical procedure.

It's essential to get in contact along with your nutritionist and get your self a correct weight-reduction plan plan that may aid you lose additional kilos. There may be an analysis course of executed earlier than embarking on any train program, which incorporates the main points of life-style and consuming patterns that may assist perceive the type of meals the person is consuming. Due to this fact an preliminary session is required so that a nutritious diet plan could be made and the person doesn't require using dietary supplements or doesn't must spend on costly health tools.

There are various elements inflicting weight achieve. It's actually vital that we eat wholesome meals as a result of our selections that we make concerning meals are essential. An excellent weight-reduction plan is a mix of various meals teams which are mixed collectively to fulfill all of the physique necessities. The meals that we devour should comprise carbs, proteins, fat, nutritional vitamins, minerals and fiber. We will get these meals teams from oats, rice and potatoes. Cereals, greens and fruits these have phytochemicals, enzymes and micronutrients are part of important for a nutritious diet. The fat may be utilized from the mono and poly-saturated meals sources relatively than the animal fat. Fats should be in small parts and have to be restricted in order to lower the portion dimension. Consuming extra of carbonated drinks on a regular basis also can end in gaining a number of weight. Different components that end in inflicting weight acquire are genetics, overeating, age, and so forth.

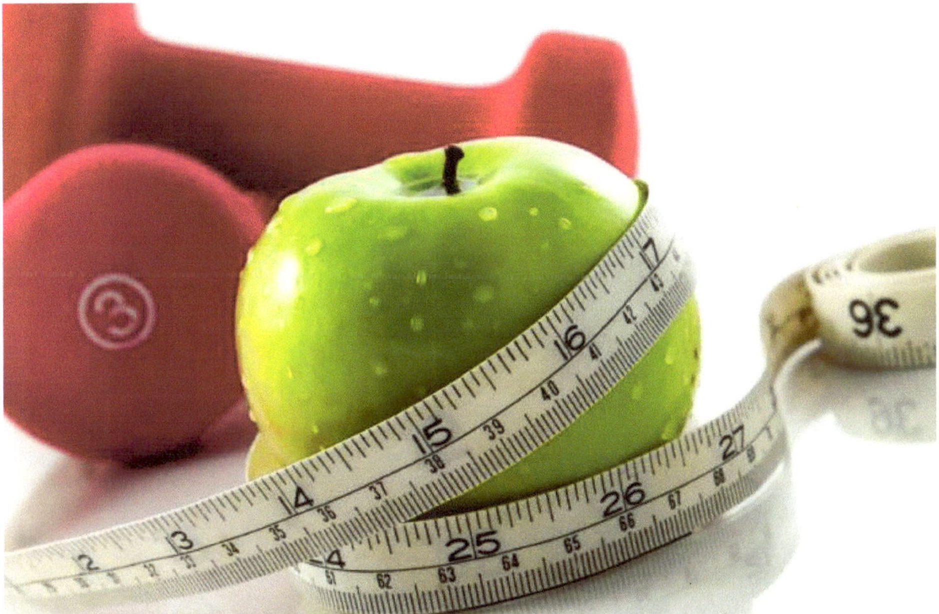

There are tons of fad diets out there that guarantees to burn fats in report time. They not solely fail to fulfill their guarantees however are unhealthy too. A few of these diets declare – eat solely bananas for per week and you'll lose 10 kilos, drink cabbage soup for a month and you'll lose 5 kilos. The claims of fad diets are fascinating to say the least. Do you ever trouble to recollect the meals pyramid that you simply studied at school time? That's the foundation of wise vitamin.

**On the base of the pyramid are carbohydrates- rice, wheat and bread. Subsequent comes greens and fruits adopted by meat, nuts, eggs and the milk group. Whether or not an individual has six or eight servings relies upon upon numerous components. The one rule is to make sure that you get not less than 1200 energy a day. The sugar consumption have to be stored at a most and fats consumption have to be stored at 20 of the full energy.**

If you end up on a energy deprivation food regimen that doesn't embody train you shed weight extraordinarily quick. It's because your physique is burning protein for vitality. Protein incorporates half the energy that fats does, so that you double the quantity to maintain the identical ranges of exercise. Apart from protein, muscle is 4-fifths water. That reduces the amount of vitality derived by one other one-fifth.

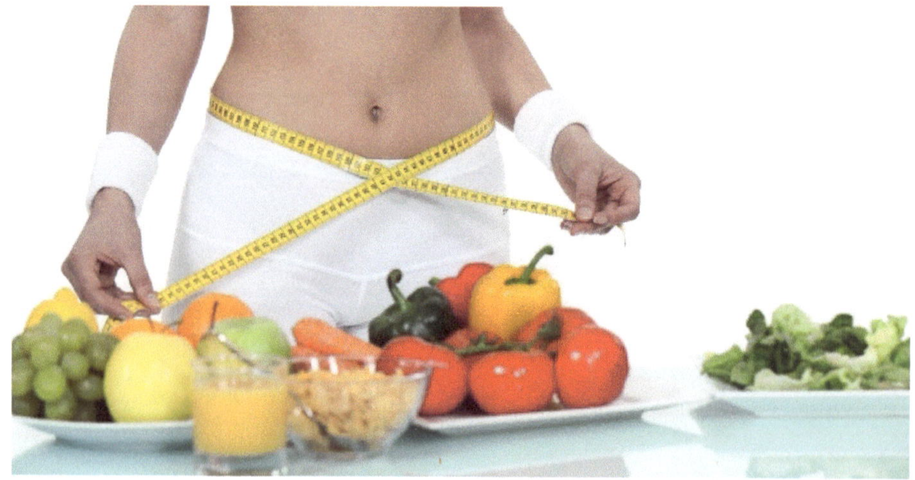

*Naturally the weighing scales appear a lot friend-lier! Sadly, by burning muscle protein the individual involved is reducing your basal metabolic charge because of which you'll burn a lot much less energy for the actions of each day residing like sleeping or respiration. Whenever you return to your regular consuming sample, the burden will come again with a vengeance, as a result of your physique is now a lot much less adept at burning energy.*

To actually see outcomes you would want to train at the least 5 days per week for 30 to forty five minutes at a reasonably brisk tempo. You also needs to get into some power coaching. That means you'll construct lean muscle mass and each pound of muscle constructed burns 35 further energy a day! You shouldn't cease exercising after getting reached your goal weight – it is advisable carry on a upkeep schedule of about half-hour three to 4 instances per week.

**<u>Disclaimer:</u>** This text shouldn't be meant to offer well being recommendation and is for common info solely. All the time search the insights of a professional well being skilled earlier than embarking on any well being program.

## The Worth of a Wholesome

## Breakfast For Weight Loss

The very first thing that folks about to begin with a weight reduction weight loss plan often need to know is, how essential is breakfast actually. This text solutions that query, and covers the perfect meals gadgets that may be part of your wholesome breakfast for weight reduction.

How vital is a wholesome breakfast for weight reduction? It is among the mostly requested questions as regards to well being and weight reduction. Nevertheless, there is no such thing as a ambiguity to the reply - a wholesome breakfast is essential to your weight reduction weight loss plan.

## Mild Breakfast is Superb

Opposite to in style perception, it's not strictly essential to pack your self with meals very early within the day. If you happen to do not normally get up very hungry, that's okay. You may probably start your day with one thing gentle and wait a few hours earlier than starting your correct consuming cycle. Nevertheless, in case you are attempting to comply with a weight reduction food regimen and enhance your well being within the course of, this can be very essential that no matter you've gotten within the morning is nutritious.

## Drawback With Sugar-Wealthy Meals

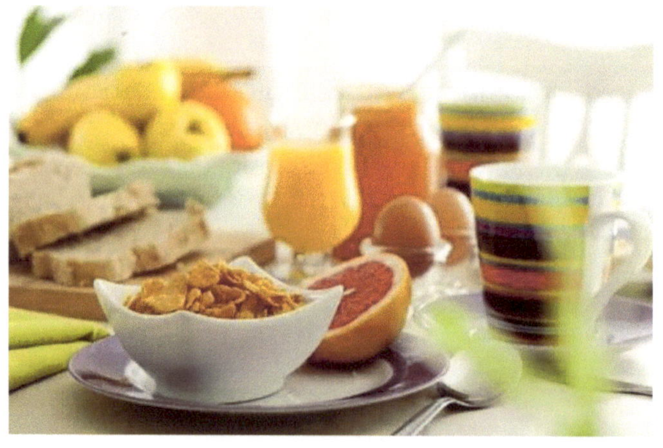

If you happen to fill your self with sugar-wealthy meals within the morning, you may be loading your self with numerous energy and 'fast launch' carbohydrates. The carbohydrates are digested quickly, which implies that despite the variety of energy you've got consumed, you'll find yourself feeling hungry very quick. This can mess up your weight reduction efforts. Additionally, within the course of there might be a rush of sugar in your blood adopted by a part of low vitality and fatigue.

**16**

## Conventional Decisions To Knock Off Your Listing

Conserving in thoughts the reasoning described above, plenty of conventional breakfast meals get dominated out: sugar-wealthy cereals, pastries, muffins, pancakes, waffles, donuts, pies and scones.

Different gadgets, comparable to common fried eggs and sausages, tacky omelets, cream bagels and hash browns are extraordinarily fatty and greasy calorie bombs that may do your weight reduction weight loss program no favors. So, what's left? Effectively, a variety of issues!

## The Proper Substances

A wholesome breakfast for weight reduction should encompass protein, fiber and complicated carbohydrates. Every of those substances will maintain you feeling full for longer and

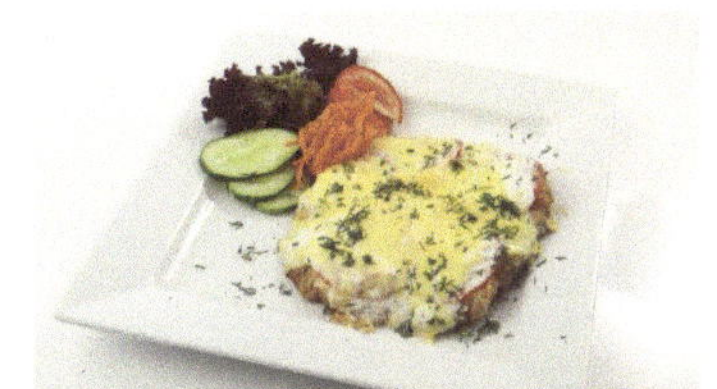

can result in extended power launch. Because of this you'll be left feeling energetic and vibrant and won't really feel the urge to overeat.

## Eggs

Eggs, particularly egg whites, are wealthy in protein, an important constituent of a wholesome weight reduction food plan. The healthiest option to have your eggs is both boiled or poached. For extra style, you possibly can even scramble them in olive oil, and add some greens, reminiscent of onions, peppers and tomatoes. Toasted complete wheat bread with some low fats butter will go very effectively together with your eggs.

## Entire Grains

Entire grains supply the proper of carbohydrates and are wealthy in fiber, which is why entire wheat bread has been beneficial above. In the event you like a bowl of cereal, a complete grain cereal akin to oatmeal, is the healthiest for weight reduction. To reinforce the style, you may prime up your oatmeal with dry fruits (walnuts, almonds, raisin) and berries or bananas. A bowl of it will make a tasty, healthful and filling breakfast that can preserve you energized all day.

## Mild Bites

In case you desire one thing mild as a part of your wholesome breakfast for weight reduction, go in for one thing like low fats yogurt with contemporary fruits or perhaps a contemporary fruit salad. Alternatively, you possibly can mix in entire fruits, corresponding to apples and bananas, with low fats yogurt and milk, for a tasty and filling handmade smoothie.

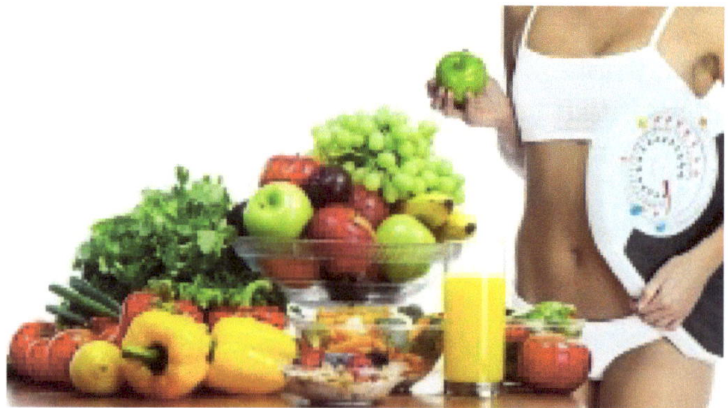

**It is humorous. Once I discuss to folks about switching their weight-reduction plan for weight reduction, most fall into considered one of two camps. The primary group tends to consider style and refers back to the dietary change with analogies like consuming shoe leather-based and hay. The opposite group largely focuses on portion measurement and**

18

**feels as if they may want a microscope and tweezers to eat their meal. So, what are some good, wholesome meals for weight reduction which might be filling and style good?**

As somebody who enjoys southern cooking as a lot as a Kardashian likes making a living only for having their image taken, switching over to wholesome, fulfilling meals that work with my palate has been a gradual course of. However, to my shock, there was a plethora of meals on the market that I like. Earlier than, I used to be simply so busy working by the crust on my fried pork chops that I did not take the time to increase my dietary horizons.

Meals like spinach, almonds, most fruit, purple beans, candy potatoes, salmon, tuna. A few of these I favored, however largely ignored. Others, I simply did not wish to strive. Now, I like all of them. And, I feel most individuals would too, in the event that they had been mixed in an amazing recipe. For those who prepare dinner, there are tons of nice recipes on the market utilizing wholesome meals that style incredible! Simply let your mouse click on away on the internet. Analysis an inventory of wholesome meals after which search for recipes which have variations of these meals and a calorie rely. Then, cook dinner and revel in.

*You could be blissful to know that even lean meats, cooked correctly, are completely acceptable in lots of weight reduction applications. So, do not fret a lot about discovering and having fun with wholesome meals and shedding weight. If this die laborious southern fried meat eater can discover loads of interesting choices, I really feel sure anybody can.*

I nonetheless have a resistance to broccoli and a few peas, however that is OK. There are many wholesome meals I take pleasure in that match my dietary and dietary necessities for well being and weight reduction. I by no means thought I'd ever eat, a lot much less like, spinach. Now, I like it! I've it for a salad base in addition to cooked and blended with different issues for a beautiful addition to any meal. Wonderful what you are able to do with the precise spices. Do not be afraid to experiment.

The listing of meals which might be each wholesome and appropriate for a weight reduction program is longer than you would possibly suspect. So, perform a little analysis and do not be afraid to place one thing new in your fork. Be comfortable!

## Find out how to Select Wholesome Meals For Weight Loss

Discovering wholesome meals for weight reduction is not that troublesome, however there are a number of ideas it's a must to perceive, and some common misconceptions that should be cleared up.

**Initially, phrases like "low fats", "low calorie" or "food regimen" on the bundle of a product does not robotically imply that it is good for you!**

As an increasing number of analysis is exhibiting, we really need a certain quantity of wholesome fat in our food regimen. Not solely that, however some meals which might be low in energy substitute sugar with synthetic sweeteners corresponding to aspartame, which may very well be even worse for you than plain sugar! This consists of "meals" comparable to eating regimen soda, weight loss plan candies, cookies and different sweets.

## Watch out for Substitutes

One other space the place it's important to watch out is in "substitute" kind meals which can be made to style like one other, larger calorie meals. The obvious instance right here can be margarine, which many individuals assume, with none actual proof, is healthier for you than butter. Margarine accommodates the worst

**20**

kind of fat, trans fat. The very fact is, since across the mid-twentieth Century, as margarine started to get extra widespread than butter, coronary heart illness within the Western world has sky-rocketed.

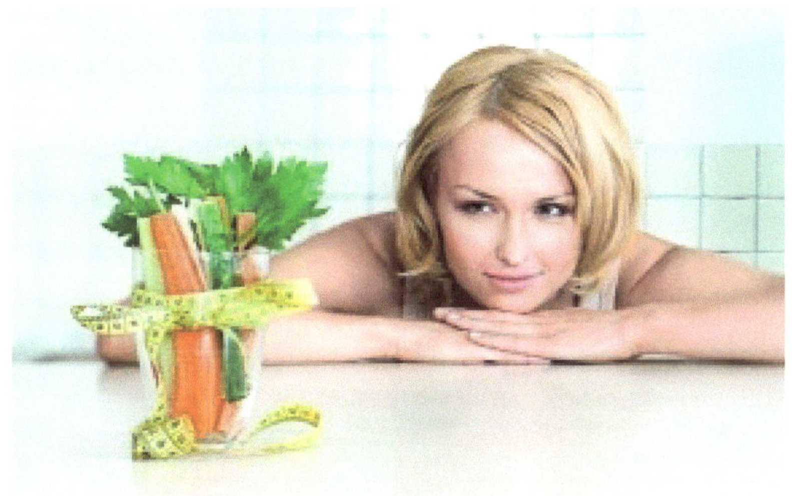

The notion that every one saturated fat, resembling you discover in butter and different dairy merchandise are dangerous is fortuitously going out of fashion. In truth, it is controversial that the worst factor about fashionable dairy merchandise are the hormones and antibiotics injected into the animals at manufacturing unit farms. The best way to keep away from this, nonetheless, is not to change to "pretend" meals, however to hunt out all pure or natural dairy merchandise.

**The Pitfalls of Soy**

The opposite frequent "wholesome" substitute for animal merchandise is soy. If you happen to go right into a well being meals retailer, fairly just a few of the packaged meals are excessive in soy. This contains gadgets like veggie burgers, tofu scorching canines, soy milk, soy pizza and soy "ice cream."

That is one other space the place current analysis has proven that consuming giant portions of soy just isn't factor. There are a number of causes for this, one of many main ones being that soy is excessive in phytic acid, which makes it more durable for the physique to soak up important vitamins.

**Soy merchandise have additionally been linked with many well being issues, together with sure forms of most cancers. Most soy has additionally been genetically modified. If you wish to know extra about this, you need to do additional analysis on the risks of soy.**

Soy merchandise which can be fermented, reminiscent of miso and tempeh are good for you, as a result of fermentation blocks the detrimental results of phytic acid. Most merchandise containing soy, nonetheless, similar to soy nuts, most soy milk and tofu aren't fermented.

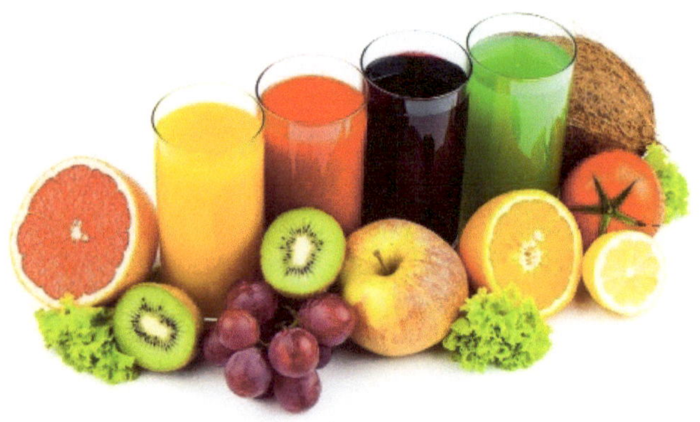

## Fruit vs. Fruit Juice

So long as we're selecting on well being meals shops, let's deal with one other favourite that such shops normally dedicate a whole aisle to -fruit juices. Whereas contemporary fruit is extremely nutritious, the identical cannot be stated for many juices. The rationale for that is that juices comprise way more extremely concentrated quantities of sugar. Briefly, you'd should eat fairly

**22**

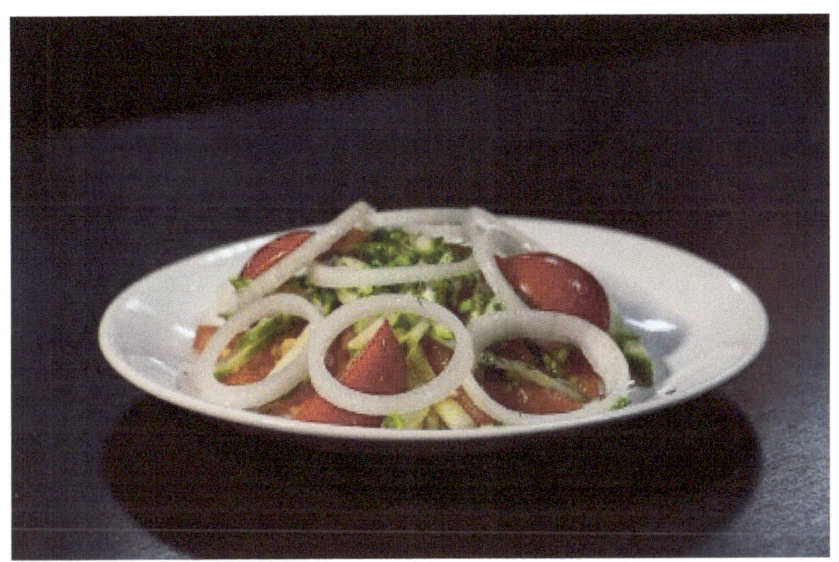

a little bit of fruit -greater than you would be more likely to in a single sitting- to equal what you'd get in a glass of juice.

Does this imply that it's best to abandon all "well being meals" and gorge on butter, cheese and meat? In fact not. Whereas pure saturated fats will be wholesome in average portions, if you happen to're making an attempt to drop pounds it is best to actually restrict your consumption of them. The purpose is, moderately, to discourage you from pondering that the favored substitutes for such meals may be safely loved.

**If you wish to transfer within the route of a more healthy weight loss plan that is additionally decrease in energy, it is best to focus much less on protein and extra on greens and entire grains. That is hardly unique recommendation, however it's one thing many individuals have a tough time doing.**

Whereas many people have cravings for carbs, meat, sweets and fat, it is uncommon that somebody craves an apple, sunflower seeds, carrots or broccoli. Once we eat these items, it is normally as a result of we all know they're wholesome and they're usually chosen as appetizers, aspect dishes or snacks.

Although it may be tough, one of the best ways to change to a nutritious diet that is additionally useful for weight reduction is to start out off with the meals you recognize are good for you. This must be finished each whenever you buy groceries, and if you're cooking (or ordering your meals at a restaurant or selecting takeout at a deli). In different phrases, do not even take into consideration the protein, starchy carbs or dessert till you've got chosen the salad, veggies and entire grains.

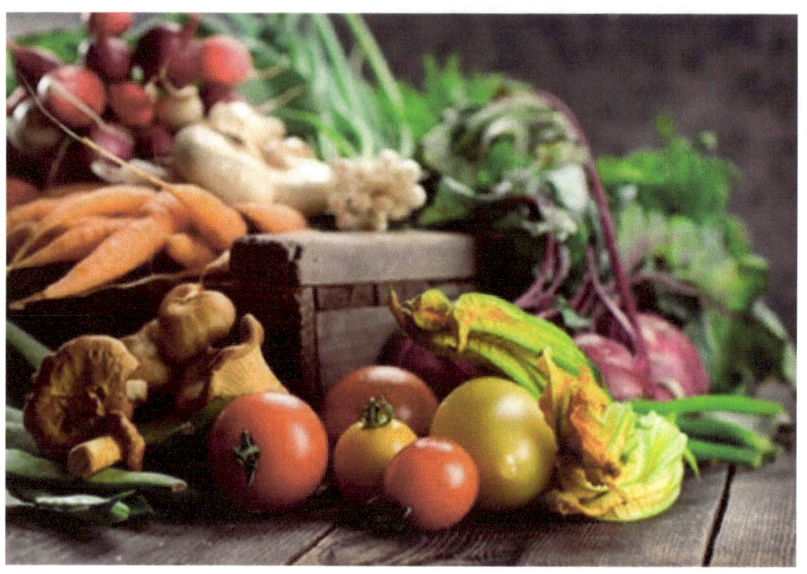

**It might appear unusual to plan your meal round a salad or portion of greens, however it may be carried out. The truth is, beginning meals off with salad, vegetable soups and recent greens is an efficient method to go away much less room for the opposite stuff that you just crave. What's good about this method is that you do not have to assume by way of depriving your self of the goodies - you will be robotically consuming them in smaller portions since you'll have much less room for them!**

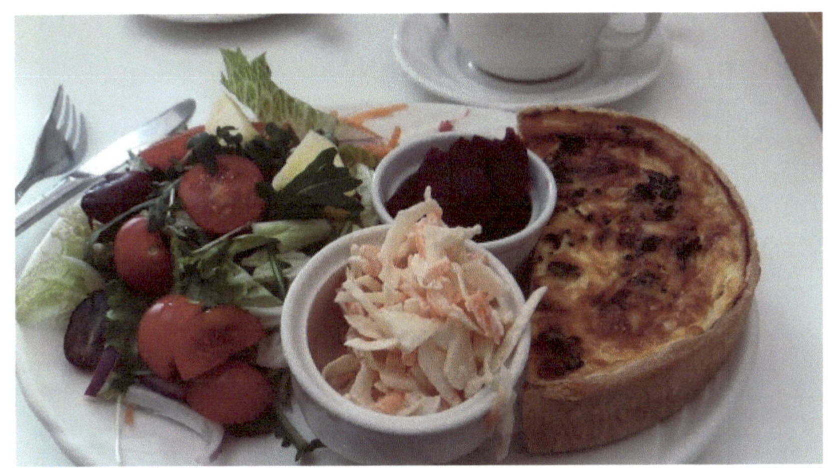

If you happen to observe this follow, your tastes may also steadily change. Not fully - you should still have an urge to feast on fried rooster, pizza, ice cream or no matter your responsible pleasures could be. However you will not really feel the necessity to take action every single day, and you will get accustomed to consuming smaller quantities of those treats.

*So, to recap, let's go over the rules we have mentioned up to now.*

*Keep away from "pretend" meals reminiscent of margarine, weight loss program meals, tofu & synthetic sweeteners*

*Eat pure or natural saturated fat, however in small to average portions*

*Eat contemporary fruit, restrict your consumption of fruit juice*

*Deal with greens, recent fruit & entire grains first whenever you store & prepare dinner*

*__Once you prioritize wholesome meals, you will have much less room for much less wholesome ones__*

Remember that these are tips that may allow you to eat in a more healthy manner, however nobody is ideal. It isn't what you do often that issues, however what you do each day. So in case you're interested by discovering wholesome meals for weight reduction, maintain such ideas in thoughts.

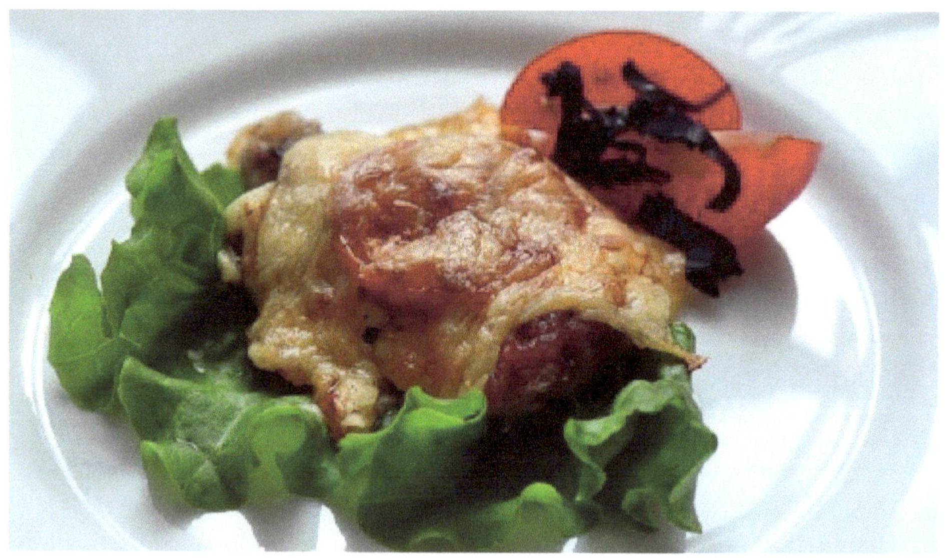

## Eight Wholesome Meals to Assist

## You Lose Weight Safely and Naturally

### 1. Garlic

Garlic belongs to one of many wholesome weight reduction meals at the moment. It lowers blood levels of cholesterol which maintain you secure from coronary heart illness. If you cannot stand garlic breath, chew on a slice of parsley after consuming.

**26**

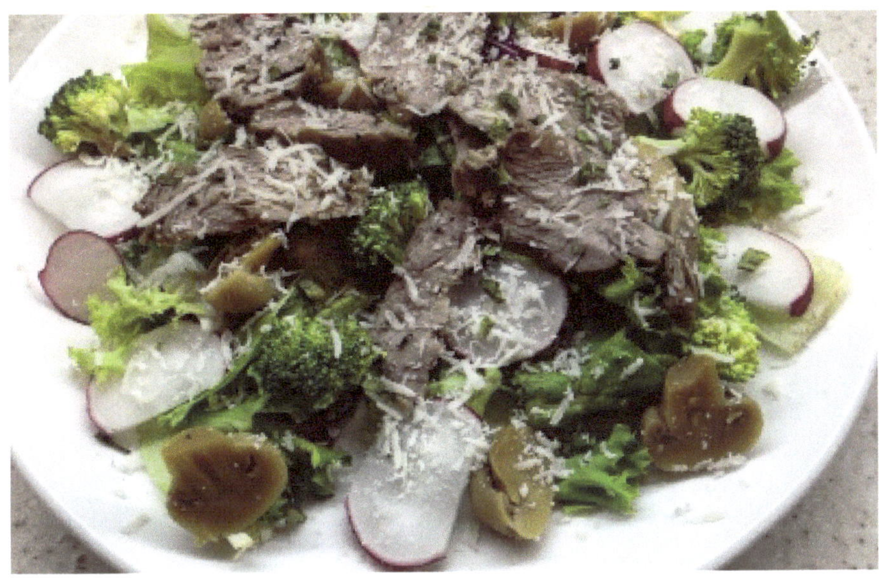

## 2. Mushrooms

Since fat trigger our bulges and different irregularities within the physique, they must be flushed out of our system instantly. By way of use of mushroom in your food plan, you may decrease blood levels of cholesterol to as much as forty five%.

## 3. Almonds

Almonds are recognized to have fatty substances. However analysis proves that almonds can really assist in your weight reduction objectives. Almonds are thought of one of many wholesome weight reduction meals due to the wealthy fiber content material it has. It additionally reduces blood levels of cholesterol which reduces the danger of coronary heart illness.

## 4. Eggs

Eggs are among the best sources of protein in a food plan plan. Many weight loss program plans use eggs due to the wealthy protein content material that retains you from ravenous. Regardless of the "yolk" avoidance of individuals, nutritionists declare that egg yolks are naturally wholesome and may maintain you away from a broken coronary heart and liver.

## 5. Flaxseeds

Flaxseeds are thought of top-of-the-line weight-reduction plan components of right now. They're a content material of many natural dietary supplements which promise to carry aid to weight reduction. They comprise alpha-linoleic acid which helps cut back irritation within the physique. Other than its anti-inflammatory impact, it's seen as one of many wholesome weight reduction meals due to the wealthy fiber content material that retains the surplus kilos off.

## 6. Pomegranates

Pomegranates are identified to be wealthy in antioxidants. Additionally they have anti growing old and anti most cancers results. They assist in weight reduction due to its skill to flush out the toxins and fat in your physique.

## 7. Purple Wine

Purple wine is probably the healthiest alcoholic drink round. It retains your blood sugar in regular ranges and it helps flush out the unhealthy ldl cholesterol out of your physique. Most weight reduction weight loss program plans make use of crimson wine served along with grilled fish.

## 8. Darkish Chocolate

Most individuals suppose that sweets make you fats. However in case you are consuming DARK chocolate, the consequences could possibly be the alternative. Due to the wealthy antioxidant properties of those sweets, the physique is ready to drive out toxins from the system. Fat, in addition to ldl cholesterol, may be lowered with darkish chocolate consumption.

## Along with this...

28

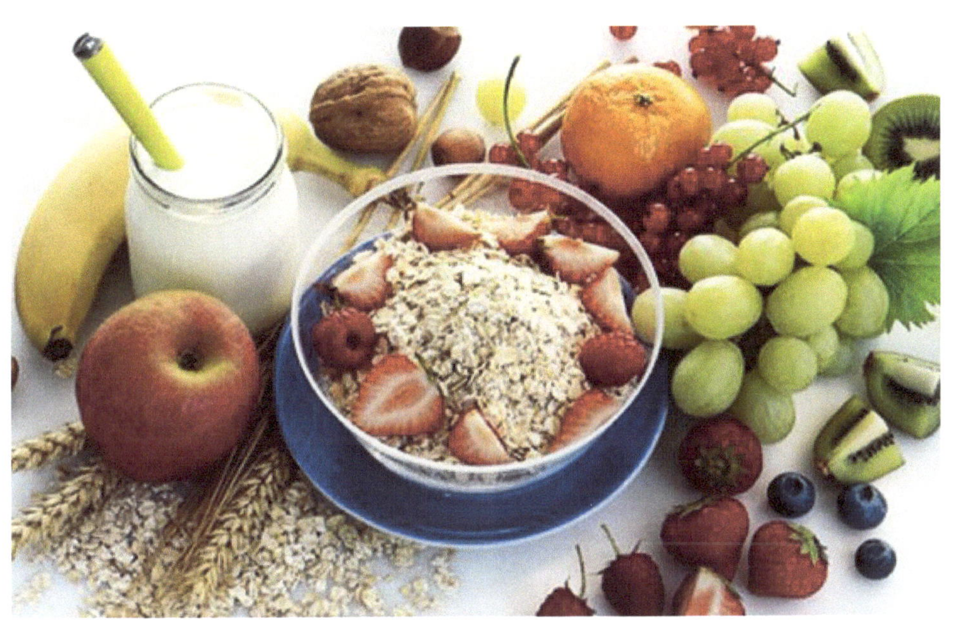

## Three Tremendous Wholesome

## Meals for Weight Loss

When you assume that meals is the enemy, you'll by no means actually have a very good angle in direction of taking your meals, and switch your plan to shed some pounds into one thing disastrous. Do not forget that meals ought to be checked out as one thing that nourishes not simply the physique but additionally the soul.

**As you savor one style after one other, it is such a pleasant expertise so even when your eventual purpose is to drop extra pounds, you continue to ought to have a very good angle in the direction of meals. In addition to, there are many meals that can truly show you how to lose the surplus kilos that you've, which we are going to enumerate within the following part.**

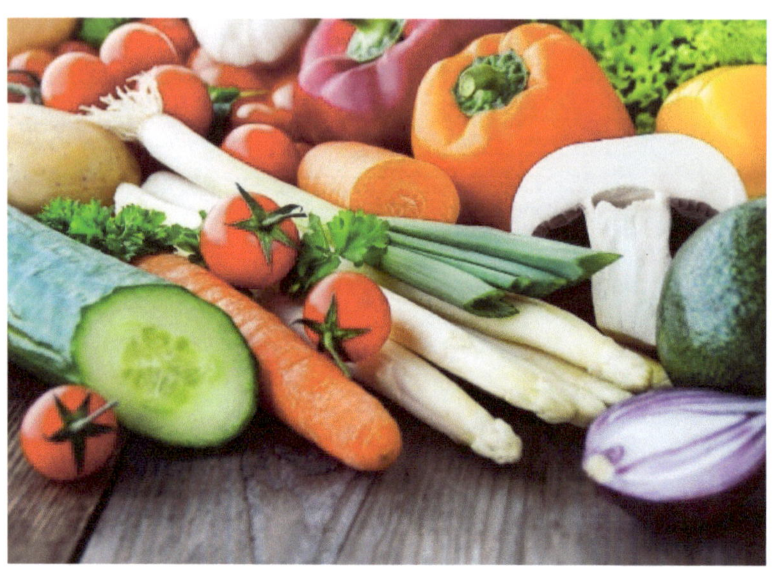

## Three Meals That May Truly Assist You Lose Weight

As chances are you'll already know, junk meals, greasy objects off the fastfood menu and too-salty or too-candy dishes are the offender to gaining weight. However what in case you handle to mix exercising with making the correct meals selections? For those who refill your grocery cart with meals that may really enable you to drop some pounds, you possibly can ultimately attain the health degree that you just'd prefer to have.

To get you began, here's a checklist of the highest three meals that may truly assist you to shed the surplus kilos that you've:

**Apples.** There's positively one thing to the dictum that an apple a day retains the physician away. Take your decide from pink, yellow or inexperienced apples and you've got a meals supply that is low in energy, sodium and is nearly fats-free. In case you're longing for one thing candy, munch on apples as an alternative of a calorie-laden dessert. What makes apples such an vital meals in weight reduction is the truth that its pectin content material releases physique fat and helps suppress one's urge for food. In addition they assist make you're feeling fuller, sooner.

**Eggs.** Eggs are a staple breakfast meals however they are often consumed anytime of the day. They are often taken boiled, in an omelette, fried or in a extra elaborate dish like Eggs Benedict. A few of the weight reduction-associated advantages of eggs embrace weight administration and muscle strengthening.

**Nuts.** One other nice snack different is nuts and seeds. A number of the healthiest nuts you can munch on are almonds, peanuts, walnuts, pistachios, pecans and soybean nuts. You can too devour sunflower seeds. All these are wealthy in fiber and Omega-three fatty acids, so you're going to get the additional vitamin whereas serving to together with your weight reduction targets concurrently they make you are feeling fuller, quicker.

**Moreover...**

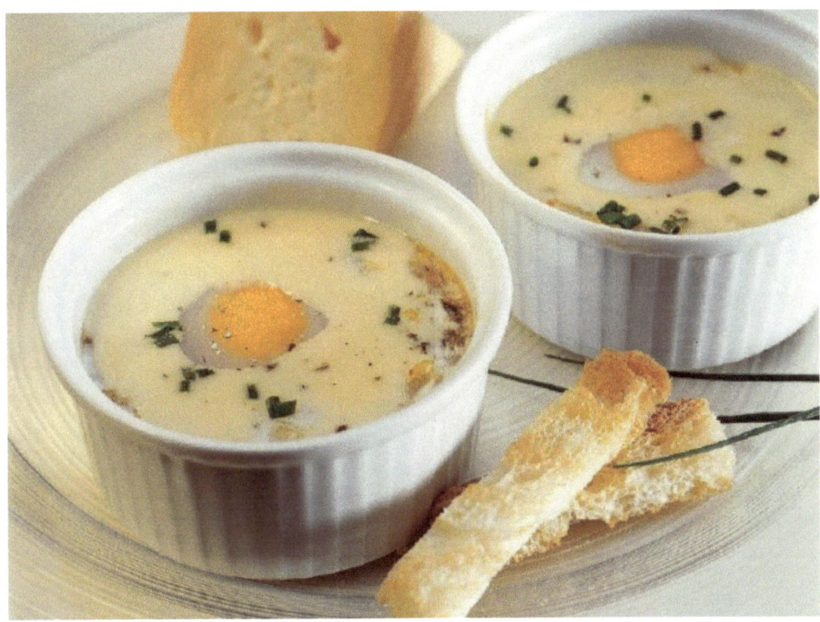

While you consider wholesome meals, do you mechanically consider meals that's bland, and never significantly interesting? However wholesome meals do not need to be tasteless! Following is an introduction to the 4 wholesome meals you need to make part of your food plan; they're scrumptious, simply accessible, and good for you.

**Beets:** Imagine it or not, beets are a really wholesome selection so as to add to your weight loss program. These small, pink rooted greens have folate and betaine, that are two vitamins that assist to decrease the blood's ranges of homocysteine. Homocysteine is believed to trigger injury to arteries and improve the chance of coronary heart illness.

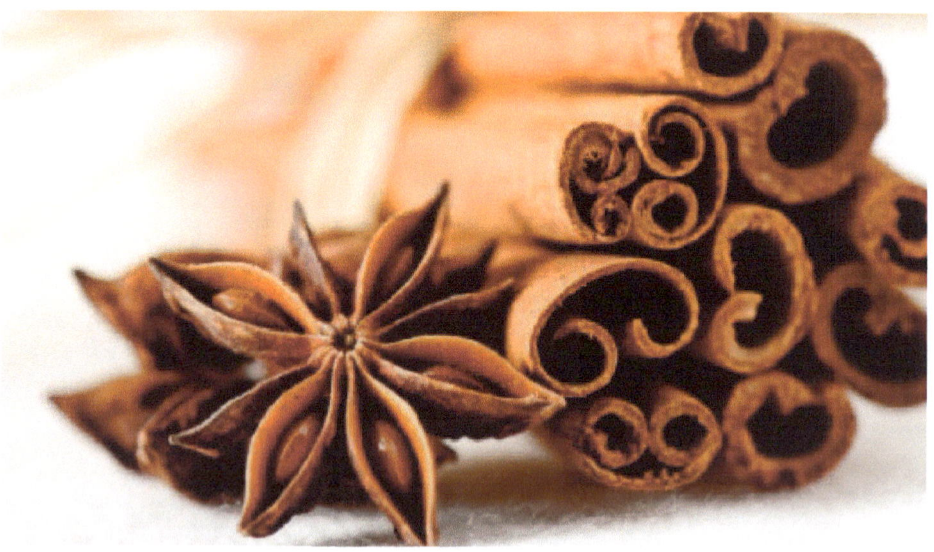

Consuming beets will scale back your possibilities of having these issues. Lab mice fed beets had decrease incidents of most cancers. Beets are at their most nutritious when eaten raw. After shredding them, soak them in somewhat lemon juice and olive oil, after which add them to your tossed salad.

**Cinnamon:** Many people solely devour cinnamon within the type of sugary cinnamon rolls. Along with being completely scrumptious, the spice additionally helps to take care of blood sugar, and decrease the danger of coronary heart illness. USDA analysis exhibits that individuals who have Sort Two Diabetes and took two grams of cinnamon per day, throughout a six week interval had decrease blood sugar in addition to decrease levels of cholesterol. The energetic substances discovered within the spice are methylhydroxychalcone polymers, which improve the physique's capacity to metabolize sugar. A good way so as to add it to your food regimen is to sprinkle it on oatmeal or cereal, or add slightly to your espresso.

**Goji Berries:** These small berries have been used for his or her medicinal properties by Tibetans for hundreds of years. Scientific research have proven that this small berry has extra antioxidant energy than some other fruit. Scientific analysis has proven the berry may also help cut back insulin manufacturing, a significant concern for sufferers with diabetes. These wholesome berries could be loved atop your yogurt, cereal, or oatmeal within the morning.

**Cabbage:** Cabbage is extensively eaten in each Asia and Europe, and is rising in popularity in America as properly. It comprises sulforaphane, a substance that's thought to cut back the chance of most cancers. It achieves this by defending the physique towards free radicals, and likewise by elevating the manufacturing of particular enzymes that forestall cell harm. Take pleasure in it by shredding it, or utilizing it to atop your sandwiches or burgers. Alternatively, strive combining it with grated apples and carrots for a refreshing salad.

# Consuming Wholesome Meals
## For Weight Loss With Little Cash

A mistaken perception with regard to maintaining a healthy diet merchandise reminiscent of natural, contemporary veggies and fruits is this stuff are expensive. Most people devour extra junk meals objects than what they want. Whereas maintaining a healthy diet to shed extra pounds could appear costly to start with, individuals should understand more healthy meals gadgets provide further benefits as nicely. More healthy meals objects typically trigger a physique to want much less quantities of meals objects all through the day. At any time when much less quantities of merchandise are eaten, then much less cash is spent.

**A physique wants protein to help with cell restoration in addition to furnish power in order that the physique runs correctly. Consuming meals like cow meat and fish present dietary protein. Nonetheless, consuming an excessive amount of dietary protein results in weight achieve since a physique tries to retailer extra protein as cellulite for future use. Even worse, consuming an excessive amount of protein is linked to diseases together with diabetes, weight problems, coronary heart illness and most cancers. As a result of purple meat and fish are expensive, consuming smaller parts could help in shedding extreme weight and scale back risk for these medical issues.**

Cash saving options to beef and fish are legumes and beans. These two gadgets possess minerals, protein, fiber, nutritional vitamins and antioxidants a physique will need to have. Canned or bagged beans and legumes are low cost to buy. These sorts of things can very simply combine into soups, salads, dips and stews. Better of all, each these merchandise have little or no toxic mercury or saturated fats, whereas crimson meat and fish often possess these horrible objects. When eating healthy to lose weight together with legumes and beans rather than purple meat and fish are cheap choices.

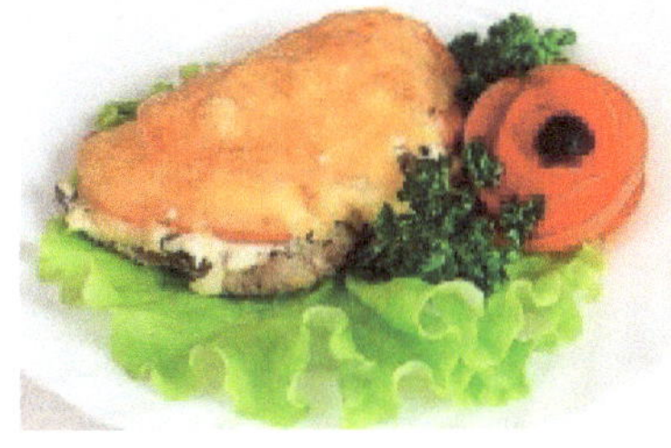

Consuming wholesome meals merchandise corresponding to recent, natural greens and fruits supplies minerals, fiber, nutritional vitamins and antioxidants the physique requires. When the human physique will get acceptable quantities of these substances, the physique will lower extreme physique weight faster in addition to decrease likelihood for medical situations. Affected by fewer medical situations contributes to paying loads much less on medical prices. This example might be yet another profit for consuming extra nutritious meals gadgets.

**Chips, white bread and cookies usually are made with enriched, processed or refined flour. This type of flour has easy carbs. Monosaccharide or easy carbohydrates digest shortly that means extra merchandise shall be eaten all day lengthy. Such meals possess little or no vitamin.**

Cookies, chips and white bread normally possess fructose, sucrose or corn sugar. This number of refined or processed sugar is also stuffed with easy carbs. These meals include no or little dietary worth.

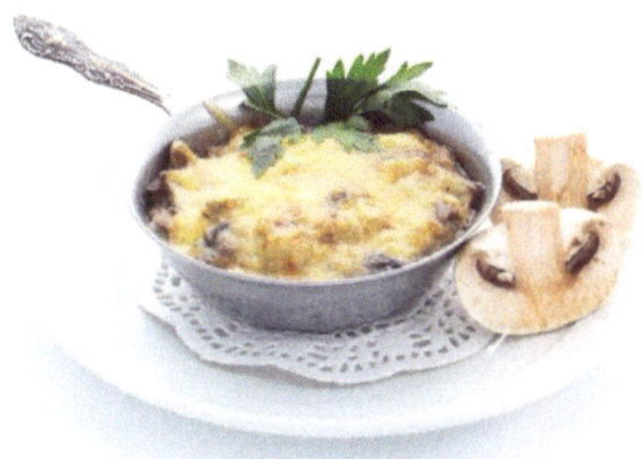

Utilizing a pair examples like chips, white bread and cookies, that are made with processed elements, reveals consuming more healthy meals could also be economical choices when contemplating the extra meals merchandise consumed and elevated medical well being prices due to experiencing further well being issues. Fruits, greens, beans and legumes comprise vitamins the human physique should have. Processed, refined or enriched flour and refined or processed sugar don't.

## Wholesome Snacks For Weight Loss:

## Sugar Is Not Welcome

Consuming 5-6 instances a day is a part of a well-liked weight loss plan to lose stomach fats. Do you ever get that feeling that one thing is inflicting stress in your life and also you hate that feeling?

Are you aware what typically occurs? You go working in your consolation zone (junk meals). Your emotional mind takes cost and sends you to the place that's good and comfortable.

It is laborious stopping the overwhelming feeling you get when your emotional mind is barking out orders to calm down and take it straightforward. In the event you catch your self, among the finest issues you are able to do is drink a giant glass of water.

It appears unusual, however you might have stopped your starvation pangs useless in its tracks with such a easy motion. If it did not work, at the least you considered slowing down your need for junk meals.

Why are you always in search of the quickest technique to lose stomach fats, when you realize it is advisable put down that sweet bar?

**36**

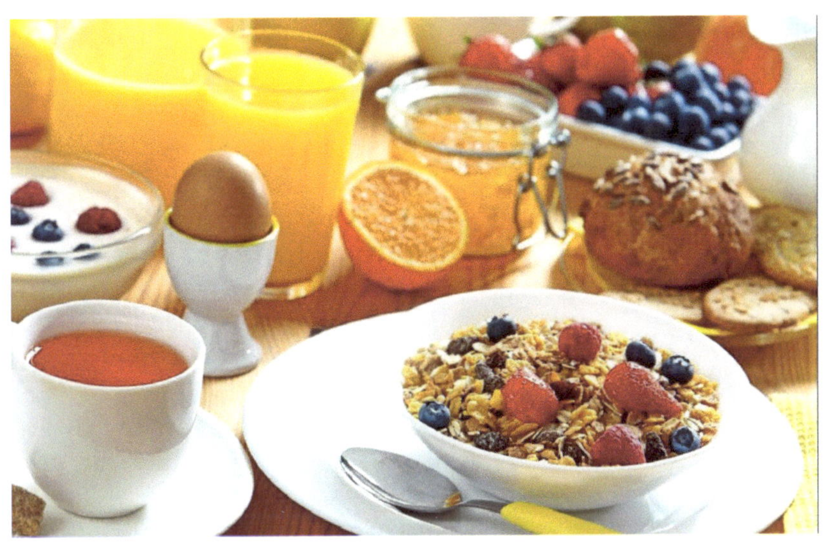

For chubby or overweight individuals, stomach fats is extraordinarily harmful. Why is stomach fats so harmful?

***Results in insulin resistance (sugar stage is uncontrolled)***

***Will result in diabetes (you do not need what comes with this)***

***Creates metabolic illness (diabetes and coronary heart illness)***

***Results in extra medical invoice***

Stomach fats feels like a humorous time period, however it's lethal severe if you'll want to drop pounds now. Sugar isn't a part of the plan to eat wholesome snacks to reduce weight.

Signs of weight problems are laborious to cope with relating to your total well being, however there are some easy issues you

**37**

are able to do. Begin by compiling a listing of low GI meals that shall be good for you.

**Low glycemic index meals monitor your sugar degree significantly better than empty energy ever might. Most vegetables and fruit are on the low-finish of the Glycemic Index chart (the nice finish). This is an incredible instance:**

**GI quantity = forty for 1 medium Orange**

**GI quantity = forty eight or eight ounces of Orange Juice**

**There's little or no distinction between these 2 wholesome merchandise, however the orange nonetheless wins. These are the sorts of choices you'll need to make about your individual well being.**

Are you able to afford to maintain chugging down the sugar when you recognize try to be maintaining a healthy diet meals for weight reduction? That is not a matter of giving up a favourite meals; that is about danger elements for Kind 2 Diabetes and heart problems.

**Successfully Lose Weight –**

**Lets Work on That**

Weight reduction program with no calorie food plan lets you shed pounds very a lot quick and that too naturally. three Weight-reduction plan applications, information for weight reduction and round one hundred fifty recipes with no calorie meals are given. Weight reduction is unquestionably a mixture of fine train and nutritious diet.

38

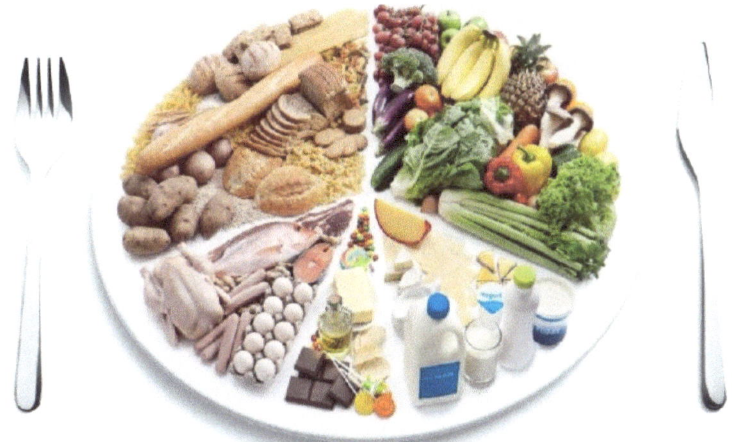

You needn't be a nut of health to lose your weight; it's important to pay full and full consideration to what you might be doing an entire day and in addition what you're consuming in your eating regimen.

**Weight reduction happens when many of the vitamins and energy are moved into the colon the place they don't get absorbed in any respect. This process of shifting vitamins and energy is used much less regularly than different varied sort of surgical procedure as a result of there may be actually a really excessive threat for deficiencies of vitamins.**

Weight reduction will not be very simple to take care of and also can enhance stress degree of a pupil and is more durable when one is affected by sleeplessness. You should be a lot disciplined, affected person, motivated whereas having weight reduction packages.

Additionally it's a must to sincere with your self. Weight reduction will not be very a lot simple as it might looks like, so I hope to make an effort to point out the components of weight reduction. Weight reduction is admittedly very a lot essential however health and well being each are developed when additional weight is misplaced and in addition train to construct up cardio and muscle talents. Weight reduction is fundamental an equation that's actually based mostly on consuming the right meals and in addition doing the proper workout routines.

**Weight reduction is many instances handled as a brief-time period purpose or a "fast repair". Until now weight reduction is a health and well being concern, which is a matter of way of life, one that may be managed properly if dealt with appropriately and rightly. Weight reduction is advisable just for people who find themselves overweight that's there BMI is far better than and even equal to 30 or for these people who find themselves chubby that's there BMI ranges from 25 to 29.9 and in addition they're having two or much more threat components.**

Weight reduction is de facto very a lot troublesome when you're feeling like that you're depriving your self. As an alternative of being thrilling and constructive expertise, reducing weight actually turns into a battle.

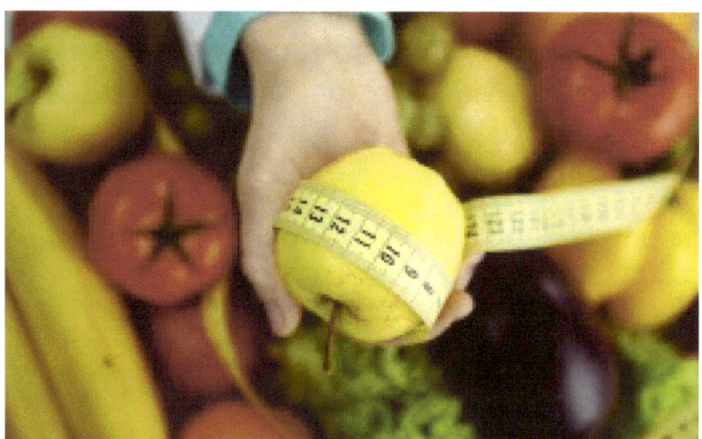

Weight reduction is the best for Group three that's the group that's utilizing the expertise-based mostly program and that too constantly and essentially the most worst for Group 2 that's the group that's utilizing the know-how-based mostly program and that too not constantly however intermittently. Because of this know-how used constantly is a lot better than expertise used

**40**

intermittently. Thus through the use of such know-how one can simply drop a few pounds and that too successfully.

## Wholesome Consuming Habits

## for Weight Loss That You Should Know

Wholesome consuming habits can have a constructive impression in your total well being situation, so the advantages exceed simply the load loss. One of many wholesome consuming habits that you will need to pay attention to is totally slicing of junk meals.

**In the case of weight reduction many individuals have to grasp that restrictive and fad diets will not be the answer to their issues. Even when they lose some kilos, they may quickly put them again on after they finish the hunger interval and get again to their consuming habits. The important thing to shedding pounds and to staying in form is to mix a nutritious diet with an efficient exercise routine.**

When you cease consuming substances that pile up and kind fats deposits and when you begin burning extra calorie than you eat, you'll be heading in the right direction to your very best weight. It's important to develop wholesome consuming habits for weight reduction and to stay to them as a result of in any other case all you will get hold of is non permanent discount of weight and a few well being issues. Wholesome consuming habits may have a optimistic affect in your general well being situation, so the advantages exceed simply the burden loss.

One of many wholesome consuming habits for weight reduction that you will need to concentrate on is totally slicing of junk meals. Attempt to eat four-6 smaller meals a day as an alterna-

**41**

tive of the classical three and embody as many servings of recent vegetables and fruit as you possibly can. Additionally work in your portion measurement and keep away from consuming very quick. For those who eat slower and take the time for chewing the meals, you'll understand that you'll eat much less as a result of you'll cease the second the abdomen despatched the sign that you're full to your mind.

**Wholesome consuming habits for weight reduction additionally embrace having breakfast each day. By no means skip meals as a result of the one outcome will likely be that you can be consuming extra as a result of you may be hungrier. As mentioned, smaller however typically meals are really helpful. Additionally watch your sugar consumption and cut back it. In case you are about to say that you do not really eat a lot sugar, simply take into consideration what number of cups of espresso or tea you might be ingesting each day and in addition take into consideration juices. Surrender fatty meat like pork and go for lean meat accompanied by a contemporary salad.**

Do not think about that wholesome consuming habits for weight reduction indicate by no means consuming out or by no means having a desert. Select mild desserts and order small parts when in a restaurant. Additionally overlook about mayo and different sauces containing a excessive variety of energy. Possibly crucial wholesome consuming behavior is to keep up your pleasure of consuming and to maintain your meals engaging. There are many wholesome recipes that you may attempt to you will see that maintaining a healthy diet doesn't have miss savory and style.

*Secrets and techniques to the wholesome solution to drop extra pounds*

Sure weight reduction packages is extra standard in a sure instances of the yr. Presumably the most effective incentives to sticking to your wholesome option to reduce weight plan is to maintain a meals diary.

**Within the pattern at this time, most American are on weight reduction downside. And the vacation season is previous approaching, many people, sarcastically, are decided to lose some kilos, earlier than we begin the spherical of events and household celebrations, the place we'll be proper in entrance of some very engaging meals!**

Sure weight reduction packages is extra standard in a sure instances of the 12 months. The primary is New Yr's, with a decided decision to lose what you gained over the vacations. Valentines Day is a further incentive. When summer time's coming and also you're considering carrying a swimsuit, it is sufficient to place everybody on a food regimen. Then, within the fall, Halloween triggers a weight-reduction plan alert. All that sweet! Oh, and the vacations are coming! You want a wholesome technique to drop some pounds that is not torture!

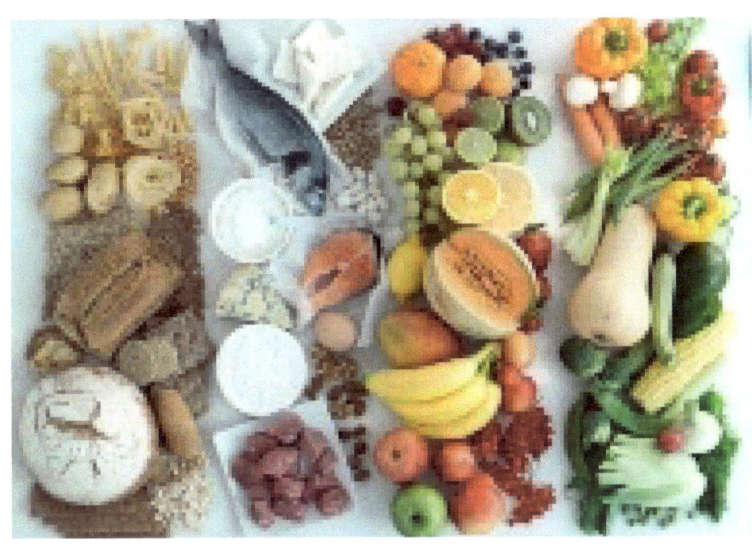

As a matter of reality, you must clearly outline what motivates you when selecting your menu and everybody has completely different causes to that. Some folks discover their garments getting a bit comfortable, and do not relish the prospect of being compelled to purchase a brand new wardrobe. Possibly you simply really feel sluggish and your weight reduction motivation is a want for extra power. One other weight reduction motivation comes out of your pleasant Doc, who cautions you to shed extra pounds earlier than you jeopardize your well being.

**Everyone knows that, there are some reputable causes. All you'll want to do is make your individual checklist of causes you're going to torture your self with a strict weight loss plan. You want that each day incentive, simply to maintain you sincere with your self. Your checklist ought to embrace as many good weight reduction motivational concepts as you possibly can provide you with and you do not wish to hurry by way of this course of!**

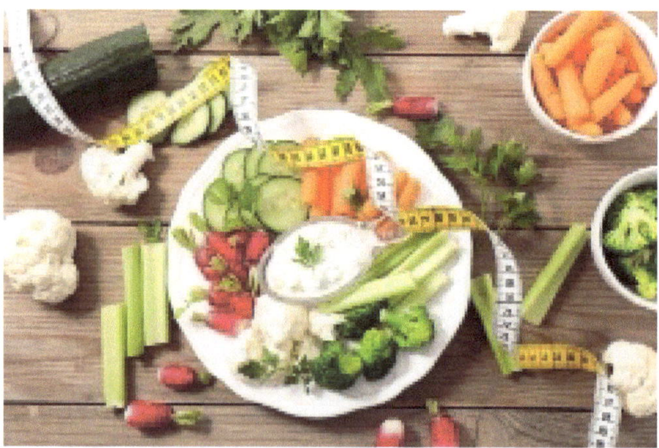

However there are some individuals strive a brand new weight loss program with every try, a few of which contain becoming a member of a membership, shopping for prepared made and portioned meals or on the very least, shopping for a ebook filled with magic weight reduction recipes. Recipes you put together from a guide usually require cautious measuring and

**44**

weighing in the event you hope for fulfillment. Right here, we will unlock the secrets and techniques of the wholesome option to shed weight and, most significantly, maintain it off! Would not it's great to weight loss program for the final time?

**Actually, one of many most important cause folks fail to realize their weight-reduction plan targets is that they really feel disadvantaged and do not even notably just like the prescribed meals. Then again, individuals who really like their meals are likely to really feel much less disadvantaged. It's worthwhile to keep on the observe with you private plan and the wholesome method to drop extra pounds. You will need to depend energy, so no matter reward you select, make it rely!**

Bear in mind, one of many traits of a wholesome approach to drop extra pounds program is that change in your consuming habits. A great way to start is to eat small, however frequent mini-meals. This provides your abdomen an opportunity to regulate to decreased consumption. Have a fruit smoothie made with low-fats milk or yogurt. This may fill you up with out loading on the energy. When you've got 5 small meals of wholesome, filling meals, you will fully pretend out your abdomen.

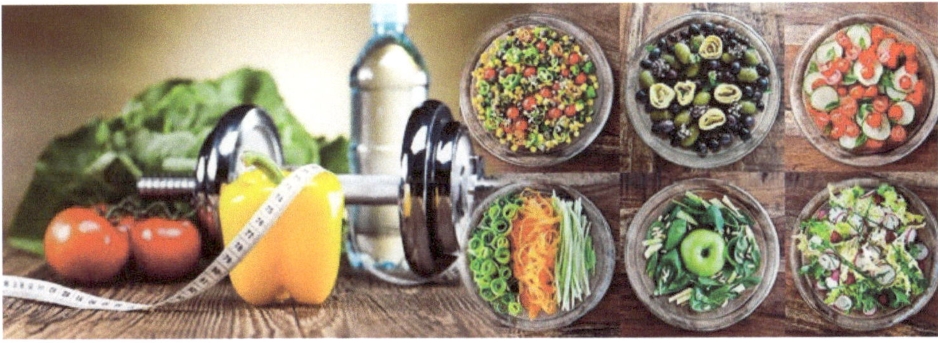

It's best to deal with your private wholesome technique to drop some weight program within the sugar scenario ASAP! Everyone knows that a single can of a well-liked soda incorporates

200 energy and a bunch of caffeine! The digital elimination of refined sugar brings fast outcomes, each in weight reduction and an improved temper and sleep.

Probably the most effective incentives to sticking to your wholesome solution to reduce weight plan is to maintain a meals diary. Write down the whole lot you eat! Log your weigh-ins, however as soon as every week solely. The meals diary retains you trustworthy and exhibits you what works and what would not. Do change into pleasant with all of the veggies you possibly can eat. I am certain you'll be taught to love it. Properly, it is as much as you, whether or not you openly tack it up on the frig, or disguise it in your nightstand. Simply go over it on daily basis, or any time you are about to shuck all of it. It will work!

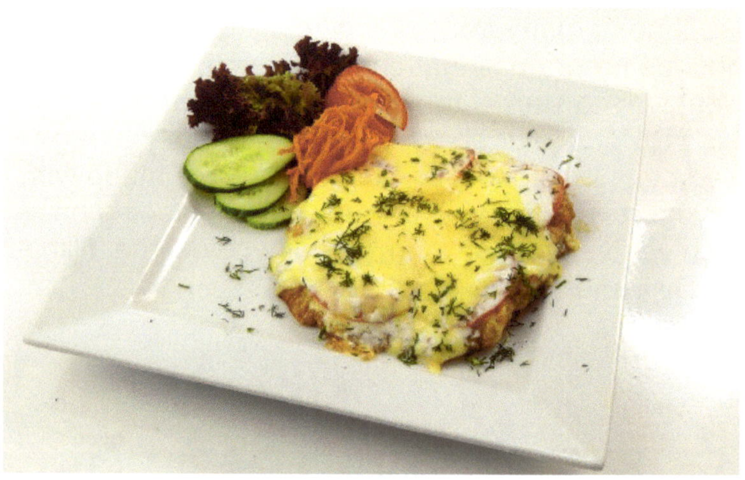

# Table of contents